Healing of Emotional Wounds

Volume 3
in the Healing Series

By Prince Handley

University of Excellence Press

Copyright © 2013 Prince Handley

All Rights Reserved.

UNIVERSITY OF EXCELLENCE PRESS
Los Angeles ▪ London ▪ Tel Aviv

ISBN-13: 978-0692230190
ISBN-10: 069223019X

Printed in the U.S.A.

Second Edition

TABLE OF CONTENTS

FOREWORD

There is nothing more vexing to the people I have counseled through the many years than emotional hurt, or to put it simply: a broken heart.

People can have physical and mental diseases, and sometimes compensate for them in their own way. However, wounds of the emotions (for example, a broken heart, rejection, scorn, loss) can be elusive.

Some people become emotionally disturbed ... some people become angry ... and some people hide their wounds by a variety of self-imposed masks.

The primal cause of this attack against your emotions – and your spirit – was not the person or people who offended you!

In this book I will discuss HOW to be **healed permanently** from emotional wounds and scars!

Healing of Emotional Wounds

Healing for Everyone

A man asked Yeshua (Jesus) to pray for his son who was mute and deaf ... plus he also at times suffered from seizures due to a demon possessing him. Many times from a child the demon had tried to cast him into fire and water to destroy him. (Mark Chapter 9:17-27 in the Brit Chadashah)

The man asked Jesus, "If you can do anything, have compassion on us, and help us." Jesus answered the man, **"If you can? Believe! All things are possible to him that believes."** (Verse 23) Immediately the father of the child cried out with tears, **"I believe. Help my unbelief!"**

ALL HEALING IS POSSIBLE IF YOU BELIEVE

When Jesus saw that a multitude came running together, he rebuked the unclean spirit, saying to him, "You mute and deaf spirit, I command you, come out of him, and never enter him again!"

Having cried out, and convulsed greatly, it (the demon) came out of him. The boy became like one dead; so much that most of them said, "He is dead." But Jesus took him by the hand, and raised him up; and he arose."

All healing is possible if you believe. Faith is a gift. Therefore, you can pray and ask the Heavenly Father for faith.

All people have been given faith. The Bible tells us "to think reasonably, as God has apportioned to each person a measure of faith." You already have a measure – or, portion – of faith. However, if you want more faith, then ask the LORD to give you more faith like the boy's father in this passage. He cried out to Yeshua, "I believe ... Help my unbelief!"

Sometimes fasting helps to bring deliverance and healing. However, Yeshua does NOT need to fast. He is God. Believe, and if you need more faith, then ask Him to help your unbelief...to give you more faith. If, however, you feel the Holy Spirit wants you to fast, then do that.

THE HOLY SPIRIT IS
GOD'S AGENT ON EARTH

The Holy Spirit, the Ruach HaKodesh, is the agent of God on earth to supply the resurrection power of Messiah. Healing and deliverance have already been purchased for you. Read Isaiah chapter 53 in the Tanakh. The rabbis never read this passage out loud in synagogue because it clearly shows that our sins are forgiven and we are healed by the stripes of the real Passover Lamb of God: Messiah Jesus (Yeshua HaMashiach).

This is the whole point of Passover: it points back to deliverance from the death angel in Egypt, and is an everlasting reminder to have us apply the BLOOD of the Lamb of God upon the doors of our hearts and homes for protection. For it is by the BLOOD of Messiah that we have deliverance and protection from Satan and his works: sin, sickness, disease, and oppression.

My questions to you today are: "Can you believe? Will you believe? Do you want to believe?"

If you **want** to be healed, and if you **believe** that Yeshua can heal you, then all you have to do is believe that He **will** heal you. **Ask** Him to heal you NOW. Just tell Him, "Lord, I believe; help my unbelief."

The Bible tells us about a woman who came to Messiah Yeshua and asked Him to deliver her daughter from a demon who was possessing her.

"Yeshua went out from there, and withdrew into the region of Tyre and Sidon. Behold, a Canaanite woman came out from those borders, and cried, saying, "Have mercy on me, Lord, you son of David! My daughter is severely demonized!"

But he answered her not a word. His disciples came and begged him, saying, "Send her away; for she cries after us." But he answered, "I wasn't sent to anyone but the lost sheep of the house of Israel."

But she came and worshiped him, saying, "Lord, help me." But he answered, "It is not appropriate to take the children's bread and throw it to the dogs."

But she said, "Yes, Lord, but even the dogs eat the crumbs which fall from their masters' table." Then Yeshua answered her, "Woman, great is your faith! Be it done to you even as you desire." And her daughter was healed from that hour." (Matthew 15:21-28)

If I put some money in your coat pocket and tell you, "I put some money in your pocket. I want you to use it for lunch today." You would probably say, "Thank you," and go on your way. Why would you take my word for your lunch money without doubting it, and NOT take the Word of God for your daily bread without doubting it. Yeshua taught us that healing and deliverance are the children's bread.

Do NOT quit, my friend. Press in for your healing and deliverance.   The LORD is faithful.

Emotional Wounds Can Be Elusive

There is nothing more vexing to the people I have counseled through the years than emotional hurt, or to put it simply: a broken heart. People can have physical, even mental disease, and sometimes compensate for them in their own way. However, wounds of the emotions (for example, a broken heart, rejection, scorn) are not only difficult to assess, but can elude instant deliverance.

In the Hebrew Tanakh (the Old Testament or the Hebrew Scriptures) we read: "A man's spirit will sustain him in sickness, But a crushed spirit, who can bear?" (Proverbs 18:14) Another translation reads: "The spirit of a man will sustain his infirmity; but a wounded spirit who can bear?" The scripture is informing us that a crushed or wounded spirit is a burden almost too heavy for an individual to bear.

SECRET REASON FOR
EMOTIONAL WOUNDS

Realize that the primal cause of this attack against your emotions – your spirit – was not the person or people who offended you. It was the devil (Satan) that used them. The enemy of your soul is NEVER fair, and NEVER honest. He likes to hurt people and lie to them. He likes to kick you when you are down.

Specific Action Plan

That's WHY you need to take your authority SOON after the attack(s) against you. The enemy (Satan) knows that if he can wound your spirit you will be defeated if you do not take decisive AND immediate action. If you have been baptized in the Holy Spirit, then **power pray in tongues** and break the attack of the wicked one against you.

NOTE:

Like to know HOW to receive this power?

Read: *How to Receive God's Power with Gifts of the Spirit*, by Prince Handley.

The scar over your wounded spirit will develop to the place of shielding the wound, thus serving two (2) purposes:

1. Protecting it from future attacks, hurts, and vulnerability; and,

2. Disguising it – camouflaging it – hiding it from view.

➡ ➡ ➡ The enemy of your soul does not care HOW he achieves this wound: through personal loss (material loss or the loss of a loved one), through demons, through mental assaults, through a friend, through a relative, through a religious person, or through an immoral person. No one is perfect; therefore, even a person who lives a normally holy life may have a moment where they slip and attack another person verbally or in gossip or in behavior.

A person can also be severely wounded emotionally through discouragement of any kind: possibly the result of a friend or loved one going astray.

WHAT IS THE ANSWER?

There are two things you must do:

First, rise up and take your authority over this attack. No matter WHAT the cause of your hurt, it is an attack from the enemy of your soul: Satan, the devil. Even if it was another person (which it usually is) that caused your spirit (your emotions) to be wounded, the source is the devil–he hates you. The other person may not even know they have done you wrong. On the other hand, they may have wanted to do you wrong. In either case, they unwittingly were pawns in the hands of the devil.

The scriptures tell us in the Brit Chadashah: "The thief (the devil) only comes to steal, to kill, and to destroy." But Messiah Jesus said, **"I came that you may have life, and that you may have it more abundantly. I am the good shepherd. The good shepherd lays down his life for the sheep."** (John 10:10-11)

Second, forgive the person or people who offended you. This is tough to do, but you have to do it. Otherwise, they are preventing or hindering your healing and deliverance from the wound(s) you have experienced. Since they have already caused you enough trouble, why would you let them bother you anymore? **Release them (by forgiving**

them) so you will NOT be tied to them (bound to them) any longer.

The scriptures also tell us: "And be kind to one another, tenderhearted, forgiving each other, just as God also in Messiah Jesus forgave you." (Ephesians 4:32)

DO IT NOW

▪ In the name of Jesus the Messiah, bind the devil (Satan) and break his hold upon you that was caused from the emotional wounds you received.

▪ PRAY and tell God you forgive the person -- or the people -- who have wounded you. Release them into the hands of God, who has told us: "To me belongeth vengeance, and recompence; their foot shall slide in due time..."

"Dearly beloved, avenge not yourselves, but rather give place unto wrath: for it is written: 'Vengeance is mine; I will repay', says the Lord."

I know this teaching is going to help you, my friend.

HEALING THROUGH RELEASE

I now want to discuss healing through release, or healing through forgiveness. Notice, forgiveness is associated with being tenderhearted. Forgiveness will also keep you tenderhearted. It prevents your heart (your emotions and spirit) from being hardened. If God has forgiven us for ALL the things we have done, how can we NOT forgive someone for what they have done, no matter how insidious or pernicious it may have been...especially in the LIGHT of eternity.

One time I was going to the post office to post a ministry mail out. While I was on my way, I was having a hard time forgiving someone. As I entered the parking lot at the post office, the LORD said to me: "Why are you letting that person rob you out of blessings? Why are you letting them bind you? Why are you letting them keep your prayers from being answered? Why are you letting them hinder you by your not forgiving them? Release them so I can bless you!"

All of a sudden, the LIGHT came on in both my spirit and my mind. I said, "God, I am NOT going to let them rob me out of blessings anymore. They have already caused me enough grief and trouble. I forgive them right now in the name of Yeshua. I release them into your hands." Immediately the LORD flooded my soul with joy. The Bible tells us: "Vengeance belongs to me; I will repay, says the Lord."

One trick of the devil is to cause people to do things wrong to you, or to lie about you, or to wound you emotionally. There is a strategy behind the attacks of Satan. One reason for his attacks as he uses other people (sometimes a child of God) is to get you angry and emotionally disturbed. Even if you are not manifesting external responses, the devil knows that if you are disturbed internally, and harbor a spirit of unforgiveness, it will keep you from the blessings of God. That is just ONE of the reasons he likes to cause you trouble.

The scripture admonishes us to "Be angry, and do not sin. Do not let the sun go down on your wrath, neither give place to the devil." (Ephesians 4:27) The original Greek word for place here used is the word *topos*, which means a place to occupy, (or, as a military term, a place from which to attack you). Do NOT give the devil an opportunity to cause you to hate those who injure you, or to cause you to take revenge, or to silently harbor ill feelings and unforgiveness.

When I was a little boy, my sister and I shared the same bedroom. One day we had an argument (probably many days!). But that particular night as I was in my bed I was angry at my sister for some reason. Before I could go to sleep, she spoke to me from her bed on the other side of the room and said, "Daddy always taught us never to go to bed mad." So we made up. That is very good advice, and even though I did not realize it then, was scriptural: "Do not let the sun go down on your wrath."

My friend, God loves you so much, and He wants to BLESS you. Do not let the enemy of God, and your enemy (the devil), trick you into being bound by another person or people. If you have been wronged, or maybe lied about with absolutely no merit to the accusation, forgive. Why would you let them bother you anymore? Why would you let them bind you? Why would you let them rob you out of blessings? Release them so God can bless you.

Picture yourself with a chain or rope tied to that person or those people who have wronged you. Forgive them and the chains and ropes – your chains and ropes – will drop off. **Give NO place (no location for**

military operations against you) to the devil.

You will not only experience release for yourself, but a freedom in your spirit, and the dove of the Spirit of God, the Ruach Elohim, will flood your soul. Blessings will begin to abound.

"And be kind to one another, and tender hearted, forgiving each other, just as God also in Messiah forgave you." (Ephesians 4:32)

I am blessed to share this teaching with **you**. Remember to **share this teaching** with your friends!

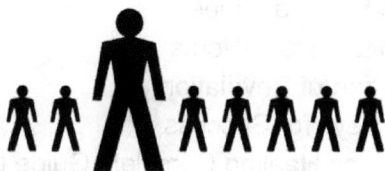

LIVE A LIFE OF EXCELLENCE

Email prayer requests and praise reports to:
princehandley@gmail.com

For a complete work on health and healing:
Health and Healing Complete Guide to Wholeness
by Prince Handley

UNIVERSITY OF EXCELLENCE PRESS

See next page for **Other Books** by Prince Handley

OTHER BOOKS BY PRINCE HANDLEY

- Map of the End Times
- How to Do Great Works
- Flow Chart of Revelation
- Action Keys for Success
- Health and Healing Complete Guide to Wholeness
- Prophetic Calendar for Israel & the Nations: Thru 2023
- Healing Deliverance
- How to Receive God's Power with Gifts of the Spirit
- Healing for Mental and Physical Abuse
- Victory Over Opposition and Resistance
- Healing of Emotional Wounds
- How to Be Healed and Live in Divine Health
- Healing from Fear, Shame and Anger
- How to Receive Healing and Bring Healing to Others
- New Global Strategy: Enabling Missions
- The Art of Christian Warfare
- Success Cycles and Secrets
- New Testament Bible Studies (A Study Manual)
- Babylon the Bitch: Enemy of Israel

AVAILABLE AT AMAZON AND OTHER BOOK STORES

For recent updates, go to:
www.marketplaceworld.com

UNIVERSITY OF EXCELLENCE PRESS

www.ingramcontent.com/pod-product-compliance
Lightning Source LLC
Chambersburg PA
CBHW060708280326
41933CB00012B/2353